How to use this booklet

This booklet has been designed to help more able people with learning disabilities who want to understand and talk about dementia.

People with learning disabilities may want to talk about dementia for a number of reasons. It is important to identify why they need to explore these issues before using the booklet. The most common reasons are:

- They have heard the word and don't know what it means.
- They have a friend or family member with dementia.
- They are worried about themselves.
- They are worried they may get dementia in the future.

This booklet is for carers to use with individuals. In exceptional circumstances, with experienced carers, it may be used with small groups of two or three individuals. The booklet does not include illustrations because we feel that only more able people will be able to express these concerns and understand the content.

Carers need to be very familiar with the content of the booklet before using it with people with learning disabilities. It may be appropriate to be selective about which pages are used, depending on which issues the person wants to explore. This may be exceptionally important if you are using the booklet with someone who is at increased risk of developing dementia.

The booklet tells the person about dementia. It describes dementia in easy-to-understand language. It provides answers to commonly asked questions about dementia. These are:

- What is dementia?
- What happens when people get dementia?
- Do these changes mean the person has dementia?
- Can you get better with dementia?
- What happens if the changes are dementia?
- Who is most likely to get dementia?
- What should I do if I'm worried that I've got dementia?
- What should I do if I'm worried about someone I know?

The Journey of life and *About my friend* booklets may also be useful for use with people with learning disabilities to help them understand the normal life cycle, and what happens when a friend develops dementia. Both booklets have large print and have pictures of a man with Down's syndrome showing how he changes over time.

Why do I need this booklet?

You may have questions about dementia.

You may have heard the word and don't know what it means.

You may be worried about yourself.

You may have a friend or a member of your family who has dementia.

This booklet will tell you what dementia is. It will tell you what happens when people get dementia. It will tell you who is likely to get it.

What is dementia?

Dementia is when parts of the brain stop working as well as they did.

When people get dementia they seem to get older more quickly. They need extra care.

Dementia is different from just getting older.

It is an illness where people have problems doing their normal jobs and activities.

There are several different sorts of dementia. The most common is called Alzheimer's.

What happens when people get dementia?

Dementia starts slowly. Friends and staff may not know at first that something is wrong.

Later on more changes happen, often at the same time.

People with dementia will forget lots of things. They may forget what they need to do next. They may forget where they've put things.

They will get muddled up. They will do things that are odd, like putting things in the wrong place.

Do these changes mean the person has dementia?

Often changes are not caused by dementia. Many problems can be sorted out.

Some people may need glasses for the first time, or new glasses.

They may need a hearing aid or to have their hearing aid looked at.

Some people get other illnesses. Doctors can make them better.

They may feel sad or worried. Something difficult may have happened to them. Talking to someone may help.

Can you get better with dementia?

No, but there are lots of things that can help.

New medicines and treatments are being tried all the time.

Some of the medicines can slow the dementia down for a short time, but they cannot stop it.

What happens if the changes are dementia?

People with dementia will become slower at everything. They may need help with the stairs. They may need help getting on to buses or down kerbs.

Some people with dementia may not be as friendly. They may hit people or shout. They may do and say strange things. They may cry a lot.

People may look different after they've had dementia for a long time. They will need a lot of help to do simple things. They may not remember who they are. They may not remember who their family, friends or staff are.

For most people it takes a long time for the changes to happen.

Staff and family will help people with dementia do as much as they can for as long as they can.

As the dementia gets worse, people with dementia will need help with everything. They will spend more time in bed and sleep a lot. Their body and brain slowly stop working and in the end they will die.

Who is most likely to get dementia?

Dementia does not happen to everyone. It is more likely to happen as you get older.

Some people are more likely to get dementia than others.

People with a member of their family who has had dementia are more likely to get dementia. Many people will be fine.

People with Down's syndrome are more likely to get dementia as they get older, especially if they are 50 or older. Many people will be fine.

People with some illnesses are also more likely to get dementia.

We can't tell who will get dementia and who won't.

If you are worried about getting dementia, it is important that you talk to your family or staff.

Doctors are looking for ways of stopping or curing dementia in the future.

What should I do if I'm worried that I've got dementia?

You need to share your worries, so talk to your family or staff.

They may ask other people to come and talk to you. This person could be a doctor, a nurse or a psychologist.

These people may want to do some medical tests. They may want to do games and puzzles with you. They may watch the way you do things.

They will try to find out what the problem is. They will give you, your family and staff the help you need.

What should I do if I'm worried about someone I know?

You need to share your worries, so tell your family or staff.

They will listen and try to find the right person for you to talk to about it.

This booklet may not answer all your questions about dementia. Your family or staff can help you to find out more, or find someone to answer more of your questions.